Hemp CBD Oil for Managing and Treating Chronic Diseases

A Complete Guide for Handling Anxiety, Arthritis, Depression, Diabetes, Pain Relief and Sleep Disorders

Jake Wood

Additionally, the information found on the following pages is intended for informational purposes only and should thus be considered, universal. As befitting its nature, the information presented is without assurance regarding its continued validity or interim quality. Trademarks that is mentioned are done without written consent and can in no way be considered an endorsement from the trademark holder.

Table of Contents

Conclusion

Introduction

Illness and disease run rampant throughout the world. We all know someone who suffers from a disease, whether arthritis, obesity, depression, cancer, epilepsy, Alzheimer's disease, or more. Even if we ourselves do not have a chronic illness, it is likely that an elderly relative does. We are also all affected by cold and flu season, which is constantly becoming harder to avoid as the bacteria are adapting to treatment and becoming "superbugs".

In the quest for better health, we end up having to go to doctor appointment after appointment, and the pill bottles and prescriptions add up. Along with this increase in appointments and pills, we also experience an increase in both the strain on our wallets and our bodies from the numerous side effects caused by the medication. Yet, there are other options available, which many of us have forgotten.

For thousands of years, cannabidiol or CBD in the form of hemp and cannabis has been used throughout ancient Asia, India, and Egypt. While modern medicine has its time and place, we need to remember that natural alternatives have their own place, too. CBD, which is a non-addictive and legal derivative of the hemp plant has been found to have many benefits, but only a few mild side effects. Not only has this powerful plant been shown to relieve chronic pain and depression, but it can even treat some of the most common diseases including cancer, epilepsy, diabetes, and heart disease.

If you are someone who is chronically ill, have an ill loved one, or want to protect yourself from the flu while promoting your long-term health, then CBD oil may be for you. Buckle yourself in, because you are about to learn amazing things about CBD and all the powerful ways in which it can improve your life. You will also learn the history and science behind this amazing plant, how to use it, how to find the best brand, and some tasty recipes which include CBD.

Chapter 1: The Science and History of CBD Oil

Long throughout history, the plants of the sativa family, both hemp and cannabis, have been used for health. While cannabis (otherwise known as marijuana or weed) may get people high, hemp will not. In fact, while the two plants are closely related and have many of the same medical benefits, hemp is approved for the use on children and is widely legal.

The first known usage of CBD for medicine originates in China, where they are widely known for their natural medical wisdom. While hemp had long been used in pottery, clothing, paper, bowstrings, and rope, it wasn't known for its medical benefits until c. 2700 B.C. At this point, the emperor Shen-Nung, known as the Father of Chinese Medicine, discovered its benefits. The emperor was a farmer, and as his subjects were frequently suffering and falling ill, he looked for a cure among the plants he grew and knew of. Legend even says that the emperor would try poisons and their corresponding antidotes on himself, rather than others. He then wrote the medical encyclopedia, Pen Ts'ao. This early encyclopedia contained a list of hundreds of natural medicines, including the cannabis plant.

While the cannabis plant was originally used to treat menstruation-related conditions, constipation, gout, arthritis, thiamine deficiency, and mental illness, more uses were discovered during the c. 100 A.D. During this time, a famed Chinese surgeon, known as Hua T'o, learned that the effects of cannabis could be utilized as anesthesia. After combining the resin of the plant into wine, he was able to greatly reduce the pain his patients experienced during surgery. Hua T'o and other physicians would even learn to use the cannabis plant to treat blood clots, tapeworms, and more.

India has a long history of using cannabis both medically and religiously. In fact, the first mention of cannabis was found in the sacred Hindu texts, known as The Vedas. The exact time that The Vedas was written is unknown, but it is estimated that it could have been written as early as 2000 to 1400 B.C. In The Vedas, it is written that cannabis is a bringer of joy and happiness and it was known as one of five sacred plants. Many of the early uses for this plant was to help people suffering from anxiety.

One of the most popular ways to consume cannabis in India since ancient times was in a drink called bhang. In this drink, nuts, seeds, and spices such as pistachios, almonds, poppy seeds, ginger, and pepper are combined with cannabis before being boiled in either milk or yogurt along with a form of butter. During wartime of the Middle Ages, soldiers would even take a swig of bhang before entering a battle to give themselves courage and relieve anxiety.

When England colonized India, they were concerned about the cannabis used by the locals. Therefore, they commissioned an extensive study to verify the safety of the plant and whether or not it could be abused. The English government was especially worried that cannabis might cause psychosis, otherwise known as driving them insane. Over a thousand standardized reviews were conducted by both Indian and British medical experts. These thorough studies sampled people from diverse backgrounds, ages, and situations.

Ultimately, after many years, the Indian Hemp Drugs Commission Report published six large volumes of data regarding the use of cannabis. They concluded that the illegalization of cannabis would be highly unjustified and that it posed less of a risk of both side effects and abuse than alcohol. They also found that the use of cannabis helped prevent the use of more dangerous drugs, such as narcotics. While these studies may have been conducted over a hundred years ago, in 1894, it is still highly relevant and holds true to this day.

Cannabis was also highly used in Ancient Egypt. Archaeologists even found traces of cannabis when they uncovered the mummy of Pharaoh Ramesses II. Ever since then, traces of cannabis have continued to be found in mummies. This proves that not only was cannabis and hemp used medically but religiously and traditionally as well.

One of the oldest completed medical textbooks ever recovered is The Ebers Papyrus, which was written c. 1550 B.C. In this textbook, there are formula recipes which used hemp to manage inflammation and pain caused by a variety of illness and injury. Some of the other uses of this incredible plant in Ancient Egypt include the treatment of cancer, vaginal bleeding, cataracts, glaucoma, hemorrhoids, depression, and other mental health ailments.

While modern history hasn't caught up with ancient history in our understanding of the amazing health benefits of cannabis and hemp, we are slowly getting there. Thanks to a little girl named Charlotte and the Stanley Brothers, they are one of the reasons we are finally advancing in our understanding of these miraculous plants.

The little girl, Charlotte Figi, began to experience seizures when she was only 3 months old. Her first seizure, when she was still a young newborn, lasted a full 30 minutes. From there, Charlotte's seizures only began to increase while becoming more severe. This continued to worsen until she had multiple seizures every day, and each seizure lasted up to 4 hours in length. This began to lead to a severe cognitive decline, and by the age of 2, Charlotte was reluctant to make eye contact and would have a violent outburst in which she would injure herself. A year later, she could no longer walk, eat, or speak. It took a long time and many doctors, but Charlotte was eventually diagnosed with a rare form of epilepsy, Dravet's syndrome.

While Charlotte may have now had a diagnosis, her parents and the doctors still didn't know how to treat the problem. Despite being on seven types of incredibly heavy medications, her condition continued to worsen. Her condition was so severe that at only 5 years old she was experiencing up to 300 tonic-clonic (also known as grand mal) seizures a week. This would even lead to her heart stopping on multiple occasions. Both the doctors and parents were at such a loss that they eventually placed Charlotte under a medically-induced coma and signed a do-not-resuscitate order. Her parents were told that nothing else could be done.

But, they simply couldn't give up on little Charlotte. Her grandfather began to read testimonials of cannabis being used to treat epilepsy and was even able to find one about it being used for another child with Dravet's syndrome. Since the doctors clearly believed there were no other options, Charlotte's parents figured there was nothing to lose by trying cannabis.

After obtaining some cannabis oil extract, Charlotte showed nearly immediate results. Whereas she was previously having 300 seizures a week, the initial week of treatment she was completely seizure-free. Once the results were clear that cannabis would help Charlotte, her parents began to look for long-term options. Her parents ended up contacting the Stanley Brothers, the owners of a rather large medical marijuana dispensary and told them Charlotte's story.

The brothers were excited to have the opportunity to help Charlotte, and they were already growing the perfect strain for her. This strain was jokingly referred to as "Hippie's Disappointment" because it is a combination of both hemp and low-tetrahydrocannabinol (THC) cannabis. Therefore, this strain contains a ratio of thirty parts CBD and one part THC and is unable to get people high. This strain contains all of the benefits of traditional medical cannabis, but without the psychoactive proprieties. The strain is perfect for medical use, especially for children like Charlotte.

Upon beginning this new strain, Charlotte saw even more relief from her incredibly debilitating seizures. In fact, the difference was so significant that the Stanley Brothers renamed the strain of hemp/cannabis to Charlotte's Web, in her honor.

Not long after, Heather Jackson came across Charlotte's Web and how it had helped little Charlotte. She began to administer the strain to her son, Zaki, who suffers from another form of childhood epilepsy, Doose syndrome.

After Zaki's incredible improvement, the story made international news and Charlotte's Web became well-known for medical treatment.

To this day, Charlotte is living a life greatly improved. Thanks to CBD oil, it has reduced her seizures to only 2 or 3 a month. She is now able to walk, eat, and talk again, and enjoys an active life. Because of the Stanley Brothers, Charlotte, and others like her, the use of non-psychoactive CBD oil has become more well-known and researched. Not only are more doctors researching the legitimizing of this powerful natural medicine, but parents are also learning how to help their children better when common medical knowledge is left without answers.

But, CBD oil is not only for epilepsy. As we mentioned earlier, ancient cultures found many other uses for it, and these uses are continuing to be re-discovered in our modern era. For instance, it is well-documented to help in pain relief, both for short-term pain and chronic pain. This is an ideal solution, as the NSAIDs (medicines such as aspirin and ibuprofen) available often are not strong enough to dull the pain of severe injuries or chronic pain. Yet, these NSAIDs also have a long list of side effects and can cause stomach damage over time. However, the option for more severe pain is still limited. While opiates are usually more successful than NSAIDs, they also come at the high risk of addiction and their side effects. This means that while people with short-term injuries will be given opiates, those with severe chronic pain are left to suffer without aid. Sadly, this leads to suicide rates being twice as high in people with chronic pain.

In a double-blind, randomized, placebo-controlled study, the effects of the safety and effectiveness of cannabis products were proven. This study is one of the most trustworthy sources, as they went to all of the lengths to keep the results as accurate as possible by using parallel groups and everything. The study compared the effects of a THC/CBD compound against a pure THC compound and a placebo on 177 cancer patients. These patients were living with chronic pain that was not managed under opioid usage. The two-week study found that those on the THC/CBD compound experienced significant improvement of more than 30% pain relief. On the other hand, both the pure THC and the placebo group did not experience pain relief.

This pain relief works at a cellular level and can greatly improve the user's quality of life. The impact is so profound that during 2017, the states which had legalized cannabis experienced a decrease of opioid addiction by 23%! The same study also revealed that people with chronic pain were able to lessen their use of opioids by an additional 64%. Similarly, states which have dispensaries for medical cannabis, such as Colorado, have found a decrease in opioid use related deaths and substance abuse hospital admissions by 15% to 35%.

Not only can the use of CBD or cannabis replace opioid use, but it can also be combined with opioids for people with especially extreme cases of pain. In the Journal of Psychoactive Drugs, one study found that when opioids and cannabis are combined, the beneficial effects are even more pronounced. This not only helped the patients experience greater relief, but they were also able to take a smaller dose of their opioid prescriptions than they otherwise would have to.

Lastly, another study during 2017 examined whether or not opioid usage may be replaced with cannabis. This study collected information from nearly 3,000 people, 34% of whom had used prescription opioids within the previous six months. Not only did a vast majority of the participants found that cannabis was equally as effective as opioids, but it also did not cause any undesired side effects. Overall, 81% of the participants reported that cannabis on its own was more effective than taking it along with an opioid prescription. Of the participants, 97% were able to decrease their opioid use due to cannabis.

But, how can CBD derived from either hemp or cannabis have such an effect not only on pain but also on many illnesses and other symptoms? While we still have much to learn about the biological effect of hemp and cannabis, we have learned that not only is it safe, but it is closely tied to serotonin.

Many people know of serotonin as a happy hormone, and when our bodies don't make enough of this important hormone, it results in depression. But, what many people don't know is that serotonin also controls many other neurotransmitters and can affect appetite, cognition, learning, intestinal function, aggression, and our ability to feel rewarded.

What is amazing is that CBD has the ability to bind directly to the serotonin receptors. Not only does CBD benefits our serotonin receptors, but it also has a positive effect on our body's endocannabinoid system. While many people are unaware of this system in our own bodies, it is incredibly important to maintain a balance of most of our biological functions. For instance, our body needs to maintain a certain temperature, specific blood pressure, and even needs to control blood sugar. If any of these aspects become out of balance, then we will experience a wide range of problems and our cells will be unable to function properly. The endocannabinoid system helps to keep all of these systems and others balanced so that we can survive and thrive.

The endocannabinoid system requires three key components to function. These are the endocannabinoids, cannabinoid receptors, and metabolic enzymes. The effects of these components are simple, yet together they form an intricate process within the endocannabinoid system.

The cannabinoid receptors are placed on the surface of our cells, and their job is to study the condition of our system. As they learn how our body is functioning, the cannabinoid receptors will send this information to our cells. This helps the cells known when and how to react to various changes.

We have many types of cannabinoid receptors, but the two that scientists are most familiar with are the CB1 and CB2. While we have these receptors throughout our bodies and they support many functions, they tend to support different aspects of our well-being. The CB1 receptors are most prevalent in our brains, and these are the same receptors that are triggered by THC to result in a high. But, the CB2 receptors do not result in a high. This type of receptors is most often located outside of our nervous system and brain and is found densely in our immune system.

Just like CBD and THC can bind to these receptors and activate them, the endocannabinoids can as well. However, the endocannabinoids are molecules found naturally in our body and are not a result of consuming a plant.

The two main endocannabinoids are molecules similar to fat, and they can be found within our cell membrane. These are produced on-demand and as needed. This means that rather than being made in advance and stored ready-to-use, they are made and used exactly when needed.

Finally, the last piece to the puzzle of the endocannabinoid puzzle is our metabolic enzymes. To keep our endocannabinoid system balanced, the metabolic enzymes will destroy the endocannabinoids once they have completed their task and we no longer require them. Whereas other molecules in our body may live longer than we need them or be stored for use later on, the cannabinoids differ due to their destruction by the metabolic enzymes.

These important aspects of the endocannabinoid system are located in nearly all of our major systems, all to maintain a balance and keep us healthy. But, because the endocannabinoid system focuses on keeping everything balanced, it is usually only engaged when it is directly needed. Whenever our body deviates from the normal, the endocannabinoid system will activate to bring it back to where it is supposed to be.

One example of this is when the neurons in our brains become overactive, the endocannabinoid system can step in. It does this because if the neurons become overactive, it can become toxic and cause damage. To prevent this, the endocannabinoid system will produce endocannabinoids directly in the brain. These will then connect to the endocannabinoid receptors and communicate to slow down.

This is helpful because the signals from our neurons usually only go in one direction. The result is that a neuron is unable to know if it is becoming overactive. But, the endocannabinoids are known as retrograde signals, which can travel in various directions. An endocannabinoid can travel backward towards the neuron that is causing a problem and directly communicate with it.

Although the endocannabinoid system benefits much more than the brain, it can also help the immune system, digestive tract, and much more. Another example is that inflammation is an important part of the healing process and the immune system. Inflammation helps protect injury, infection, and disease. If we have gotten a cut, the immune system will release inflammation to help prevent the body from becoming infected by bacteria. Without inflammation and the immune system that controls it, we would die from a simple cut or cold.

Yet, chronic disease and auto-immune illnesses are known to cause excessive inflammation throughout the body. This increased inflammation may even attack our healthy cells. This can become dangerous, not just leading to chronic pain, but causing a deterioration of our body. Thankfully, studies have found that the endocannabinoid system can help monitor our immune system, cutting off inflammation when we begin to develop too much. Because of this, researchers believe that further activating the endocannabinoid system with either CBD or cannabis, could prove to be a successful treatment option for people with auto-immune illnesses or those that otherwise cause inflammation.

But, why do hemp and cannabis affect this endocannabinoid system? This is because the CBD, THC, and other components found in either hemp or cannabis are plant-derived cannabinoids. They have the ability to function just like the cannabinoids naturally found in our bodies. This is why THC can get people high because it will activate the receptors located in our brains.

Yet, this raises other questions. If we already have cannabinoids affecting our brain, why does THC make us high? And, why aren't we constantly high from our own endocannabinoids?

Two reasons. Firstly, while the metabolic enzymes can break down our own endocannabinoids, they are not able to break down the THC. This results in the THC lingering in our brain much longer than our own endocannabinoids.

Secondly, while both THC and our own naturally endocannabinoids affect the brain, the way in which they affect the brain can slightly differ. This is because our neurotransmitters, such as cannabinoids, affect multiple types of receptors. For instance, CBD can interact with many types of receptors in our brain, rather than a single receptor. In the same way, THC and other plant-derived cannabinoids likely affect many other receptors than natural cannabinoids found in the body. This is likely what triggers the high effect.

Learning about the endocannabinoid system, it's plain to see why CBD can have such a profound effect. But, how exactly does the endocannabinoid system process CBD? There are multiple ways, and they are incredibly powerful, especially the ability of CBD to affect the number of natural endocannabinoids we have in the brain. When we consume CBD, it neutralizes one of the metabolic enzymes, specifically the one which causes the breakdown of the natural cannabinoid known as anandamide. Specifically, negating this enzyme and promoting this cannabinoid has been shown to affect mental health and protect our neurons positively. Researchers believe that this could be a useful treatment option when treating various anxiety-related disorders, seizures, and other conditions.

CBD has the ability to beneficially interact with our ion channels, which are membrane proteins which form pores, allowing ions to pass through. For instance, they can form onto a receptor in these locations, which allows for the management of inflammation, the perception of pain, and body temperature. This receptor (named the "vanilloid" receptor after the vanilla bean) is also known to unclog blood vessels and relieve headaches. It also contains antiseptic properties.

Along with affecting our serotonin and vanilloid receptors, CBD has the ability to affect a receptor known as the "orphan". The reason it is referred to as such is that scientists are still uncertain whether or not it belongs to a larger group of receptors. The orphan receptors are found densely in the brain, especially in high quantities within the cerebellum. Blood pressure, bone density, and other biological processes are controlled by the orphan receptors.

But, when the orphan receptors are overactive, they can cause osteoporosis by causing the reabsorption of bone. They have even been shown to promote the growth of cancer cells for multiple types of cancer. Thankfully, studies have shown that by blocking the orphan receptors with CBD, we may be able to reduce both osteoporosis and cancer growth.

However, this is not the only way in which CBD can inhibit cancer growth. By activating certain receptors (known as PPARs), the CBD can directly shrink the size of certain tumors, especially in lung cancer. By activating this same receptor, CBD is also able to reduce the risk of Alzheimer's disease, balance insulin, and increase energy, among other benefits.

A group of Australian scientists was able to learn that CBD has the ability to alter the shape of the GABA-A receptor. This process helps increase the binding affinity of the receptor and increases the natural calming effects of GABA. Increasing the effectiveness of GABA could help similarly to medications such as Valium, Xanax, and other calming drugs in the benzodiazepine family.

Lastly, unlike THC, CBD will not lead to a high. This is because CBD is unable to bind to the same receptors directly. Yet, it can change the shape of these receptors to make THC more effective. This is beneficial for people who want to use CBD medicinally, as even if they choose a product with moderate amounts of THC, they are unlikely to get high. Though, depending on the ratio of THC to CBD, it is possible to get high off of cannabis that contains a high CBD content. For this reason, most

CBD products are made with hemp, which contains such a small amount of THC that it is legal in most places and unable to cause a high.

THC and CBD have been shown to be more effective together, although CBD is still extremely powerful on its own. And, by using hemp CBD products you are able to receive the numerous benefits of CBD without the THC caused high. Even without THC, CBD is known to increase mental health, protect the brain, prevent seizures, shrink cancer cells, manage pain, and more.

While the effects of the plant-derived cannabinoids on our cannabinoid system are profound, this is not the only way in which both hemp and cannabis can benefit our health. Another powerful aspect of these plants lies in their terpenes. In fact, terpenes are found in many plants and are frequently used for their natural healing properties. You may be wondering what these powerful terpenes are. Put simply, they are the molecules found in plants that result in their rich aroma, color, and flavor. The plants which have stronger scents tend to have a higher terpene content. For example, lavender, orange, rosemary, and camphor are all plants high in terpenes that are used for their medical benefits.

All of these plants contain various terpenes. For instance, lavender is high in the terpene linalool. This terpene is what gives lavender its calming and anti-anxiety effects. In the same way, both hemp and cannabis contain terpenes which can have their own benefits, depending on the species and which terpenes it contains. Brands will often even name their products after the terpenes that are within them.

For example, Lemon Kush is named so because of the

terpenes in it cause it to have a lemon aroma and flavor.

In fact, people often become attached to certain strains of hemp or cannabis, depending on the flavor and scent it has from its terpenes. They can have a wide depth of both health benefits and sensory experience, as the cannabis and hemp plants contain over 100 to 200 types of terpenes. While each plant will contain a slightly varying number of terpenes, the ones it does contain will work synergistically well with one another.

While terpenes are different from cannabinoids, they benefit us in a similar way. They can bind to our cannabinoid receptors, which can give us certain benefits. This means that if you want a specific benefit, such as a strain that will help with anxiety, you can try to find a brand of CBD that also contains the terpene linalool. Knowing about the most common terpenes and their effects can better help you target your individual symptoms and increase the benefits you experience.

Linalool

Well-known for being found in lavender, hops, and basil, linalool contains a mainly floral aroma, but with some spicy overtones as well. The main benefits of linalool are anti-epileptic, anti-inflammatory, antidepressant, antipsychotic, anti-anxiety, calming, and pain relieving.

Pinene

Also known as a-pinene or alpha-pinene, this is the most commonly occurring terpene found in plants And, as you probably guessed, pinene is famous for the flavor and scent of pine. This terpene can help many people with lung illnesses such as asthma because it is a bronchodilator. Pinene is also anti-inflammatory, antioxidant, antibacterial, reduces the growth of cancer cells, and relieves pain.

Limonene

Often found in citrus, limonene is especially powerful because it increases the absorption of terpenes both through the mucous membranes and the skin. Other benefits including it being an anti-inflammatory, anti-fungal, an anti-depressant, as well as reducing the growth of cancer cells, calming the body and mind, reduces acid reflux, increases the immune system, and reduces pain.

Terpineol

Terpineol is naturally found in over 150 types of plants. Yet, it can sometimes be difficult to detect as it often goes hand-in-hand with pinene, which may often overpower the terpineol. This terpene can often be found in lilacs, lime blossoms, eucalyptus, and pine. While terpineol is most known for its relaxation effect, it is also an anti-inflammatory, antibiotic, anti-anxiety, and anti-tumor terpene.

Myrcene

While the molecules for myrcene are some of the smallest of all the terpenes, it is the most prevalent variety found in cannabis. This terpene is more likely to be found in indica strains; these strains cause a deeply relaxing and sedative effect that myrcene is known for. Myrcene is also highly concentrated in mango, lemongrass, and hops. Some of the benefits you can experience from this terpene include anti-inflammatory, antibacterial, anti-psychotic, anti-spasmodic, anti-diabetic effects, as well as the shrinking of cancer cells and pain relief.

Caryophyllene

Commonly found in spices such as cinnamon, cloves, and black pepper, caryophyllene is characterized by its spicy aroma. It can also be found in high quantities in rosemary, basil, oregano, and hops. This terpene is especially powerful on the cannabinoid receptor CB2, meaning it is a powerful anti-inflammatory. For this reason, it is often put into salves for pain relief and injuries. Caryophyllene is also known to lessen cancer growth, protect neuron health, reduce anxiety and depression, kill bacteria, and reduce pain.

Bisabolol

While bisabolol has long been used in the cosmetic industry, it has only recently been under research for medical use due to its benefits found in cannabis. This terpene, also known as levomenol, is most often found in chamomile and has a light and sweet floral aroma. Bisabolol is well-known to fight against acute leukemia cells, and it also has anti-inflammatory, antimicrobial, and anti-irritant properties.

Humulene

Humulene is characterized by its woody and slightly earthy scent which is accented with spicy notes. It can commonly be found in clove, basil, and hops. Though people often associate the munchies with cannabis, humulene is largely known to suppress hunger. Humulene is also known to be anti-inflammatory, antibacterial, and contains pain relieving properties as well.

Ocimene

Naturally found in orchids, parsley, mint, basil, pepper, kumquats, and mangoes, ocimene contains a sweet, pleasant aroma which is slightly woodsy and is often utilized in perfume. Ocimene is well-known to have anti-fungal, antiviral, antiseptic, antibacterial, and decongestant effects.

Valencene

While the benefits of valencene are still being researched, it appears to have anti-inflammatory benefits. It is also a well-known insect repellent. This terpene is commonly found in oranges, tangerines, and grapefruit, and is often the reason for a sweet citrus aroma in cannabis and hemp.

Geraniol

Also known as lemonol, geraniol is most well-known for the distinct and delicate scent it presents within geranium blossoms. Though, as its alternative name suggests, it can also be found in lemons, and even in tobacco. The scent and flavor often remind people of citronella candles, but it may remind others of passion fruit, stone fruits, or roses. Some of the benefits of this terpene are that it helps stop tumor cell growth, protects the brain from disease and injury, and acts as an antioxidant, antibacterial, antiviral, anti-fungal, and an antispasmodic.

Terpinolene

Known for its sedative properties, terpinolene is also an antioxidant, antibacterial, and anti-fungal. It can even help prevent insomnia and top the growth of cancer cells. This terpene is commonly found in lilacs, conifers, apples, nutmeg, and cumin.

Borneol

Most known for being in camphor, borneol has been used for thousands of years in Chinese medicine. While this terpene can help with insomnia, it is especially beneficial for pain. In fact, studies have shown that it can decrease pain and inflammation so much that it may be able to replicate lidocaine when applied topically.

Eucalyptol

While most known for being in eucalyptus, this terpene can also be found in sweet basil, tea tree, camphor, bay leaves, sage, rosemary, and more. Eucalyptol is a powerful decongestant and can greatly help those with asthma or cough. Eucalyptol also has anti-inflammatory, antioxidant, antibacterial, and anti-viral properties. Along with relieving pain, protecting against Alzheimer's disease, and stopping the growth of cancer cells.

BCP

BCP (Beta-Caryophyllene) was only recently discovered as an active compound within cannabis and hemp. But, it can bind to the cannabinoid receptors to greatly reduce inflammation and pain. It can also be found in cloves, cinnamon, rosemary, lavender, basil, oregano, and ylang-ylang. BCP has also been found to help relieve anxiety, promote digestion, and boost the immune system. This terpene is considered one of the most beneficial compounds within cannabis. For this reason, the FDA has approved the non-psychoactive BCP as a dietary supplement.

As you can see, there are many compounds and molecules that go into both hemp and cannabis for it to have its many benefits. While there is still much that needs to be learned about these compounds, science has well-established that it is safe and can help treat various ailments in many ways. Having this basic understanding of CBD, hemp, cannabis, and terpenes will allow you to use CBD oil more effectively and better know which brand is best for you as an individual.

Chapter 2: The Benefits of CBD and How to Use it to Manage Illness

The reasons for choosing CBD oil are clear. Not only is it an effective and powerful treatment option, but it is also affordable and has a few negligible side effects. While this can benefit people worldwide, it is especially helpful in America where illness is skyrocketing while the rates of insured people are decreasing. In fact, a study from 2017 found that over 30% of millennials have to refuse medical aid because they simply can't afford it. Even many of the people who have health insurance still can't afford treatment with it due to the high copays and deductibles.

If that wasn't bad enough, the price of prescription drugs has exorbitantly increased while the minimum wage and average salaries have generally remained the same. In fact, this problem is so severe that many of the most well-known and prescribed prescription drugs have been increased in price by nearly ten times the inflation rate.

This problem is well-illustrated by Pfizer Inc. This company is one of the largest producers of prescription drugs in America. During 2016, Pfizer Inc. raised their prices on over 130 of their products. Nearly all of the price increases were 10% higher than what the price had previously been.

While medical care is speedily increasing in price leaving people without care, the statistics on chronic illness are also grim.

Cancer is as big of a problem as ever, and one study even estimates that 2018 will experience over 1.7 million new cases of cancer and over 600,000 deaths caused by this devastating disease in America alone.

Another study found that an estimated 3.4 million people have epilepsy which is currently active. Of these millions of people, nearly 500,000 are children.

Sleep disorders, which are known to raise the risk of disease and early death, are on the rise as well. These include illnesses such as sleep apnea, insomnia, night terrors, and narcolepsy. They affect up to 70 million people in America.

Physical illnesses are not the only ones on the rise; mental illness is affecting even more Americans as well. Anxiety disorders are extremely common and affect 40 million adults alone. Major depressive disorder is also on the rise, increasing cases of suicide. This condition, which leaves the person feeling as though they are unable to keep on living, is affecting an average of 16.1 million adults.

Finally, chronic pain leaves a person barely able to cope in life. Many people are permanently disabled and unable to get out of bed due to severe pain. This condition affects over 11% of Americans, with 25.3 million people suffering from it daily. Of these people living with chronic pain, over 23 million experience extreme pain regularly.

While people are currently suffering from a lack of healthcare and an increase in illness, they are also suffering from being unable to get the care they need even if they can afford it. Due to the rise of opioid-related deaths (mostly from people who illegally bought it off the street), there has been a movement to decrease the prescription of opioids. While this movement comes from a good place in peoples' hearts and is essential, it is also important to acknowledge chronic pain patients. Chronic pain is often so severe that people are unable to cope, and many end up taking their own lives if they are unable to get their pain relieved. This problem is so severe that the rates of suicide twice as high for people who live with chronic pain. Restricting pain medication from these people is not only inhumane, but it also increases their death rates.

Thankfully, CBD oil has been shown to help aid in the treatment and management of all of the illnesses I just mentioned. Many studies have proven its effects on severe pain, epilepsy, sleep disorders, cancer, and more. Not only that, but CBD is much more affordable than many prescription drugs with a fraction of the side effects. A 2017 study even found that CBD oil is much easier for patients to remain using long-term than the previous prescription drugs they had been on, thanks to the lack of side effects and the effectiveness of CBD. The side effects are usually minimal, and most people don't even experience them. These negligible side effects include slight diarrhea, tiredness, and changes in weight or appetite when people consume large doses.

Whether you are living with a physical condition, neurological disorder, mental illness, or simply want to improve your health, CBD may be the answer. Science has well-shown its many benefits, and it has been proven that these are not false promises. CBD may not be for everyone, but if you never give it a try to won't know what you are missing out on. The effects of this oil are powerful and have the ability to help many people from various lifestyles and with many different illnesses.

Arthritis

While both rheumatoid arthritis and osteoarthritis are different, both are characterized by severe degenerative pain and swelling in the joints. Rheumatoid arthritis is an autoimmune disease caused when a person's immune system attacks their joints. Osteoarthritis is a degenerative disease which is caused when the cartilage in a person's joints degrades over time. Thankfully, CBD has been found to not only relieve the severe pain these illnesses cause, but it could even help manage the conditions themselves.

In a controlled study on CBD's effects on rheumatoid arthritis, it was found that not only did it significantly reduce the participants' pain, but it also greatly reduced the progression of the autoimmune disease.

The current methods of treatment for osteoarthritis are greatly limited, as there are no drugs on the market that can reduce the progression of the disease and the pain management options are greatly limited. However, preclinical studies have found that utilizing the endocannabinoid system could possible directly target the disease. The evidence suggests that not only could CBD block or greatly reduce the pain caused by the illness, but it might even slow the development of the disease and prevent nerve damage in the joints.

One of the great things about CBD is that you can consume it in food, place drops of the oil under your tongue, vape it, or even apply it topically. This is good news for arthritic patients because they can both consume some for full-body benefits, but also apply it topically to the joints that are causing the most pain.

Depression

While most people who don't suffer from mental illness typically assume that depression is someone feeling sad, it is much more than that. In fact, depression can make it difficult for people to feel any feelings at all. Yet, when they are able to experience emotions, they often feel miserable and possibly even hatred for themselves. It becomes hard to stay alive and even if you don't want to die.

Depression can come in many forms: persistent depressive disorder, seasonal affective disorder, postpartum depression, and major depressive disorder. But, they all share the commonality that they really make a person suffer simply by being awake. In fact, depression is one of the leading causes of disability for people ages 15 to 44. This is especially serious because two-thirds of people with depression never seek help or receive treatment. This results in suicide being a leading cause of death for people ages 15 to 44.

While medication may help some people, it's a long and difficult process of trial and error for many, unable to find anything that helps them. Thankfully, CBD may be able to help these people. CBD has the ability to affect our limbic system and hippocampus in our brains, which is what affects our emotions, hunger, and other functions. It can also help heal our neurons and increase serotonin levels.

In a study conducted in 2006, it was found that the use of cannabis was able to decrease depressive symptoms and episodes compared to those who did not use the plant. Another study found that CBD can reduce anxiety and stress, which often worsened by depression.

Along with the studies showing the benefits of CBD on depression, there is ample anecdotal evidence and testimonials. Thanks to CBD, some people may not need antidepressants anymore, while others may find that CBD paired with their antidepressants help them have better control. Either way, CBD can be a wonderful addition to your mental health and self-care protocol.

Diabetes

For those people with diabetes, depending on if they live with type I or type II, the pancreas is either unable to utilize insulin sufficiently to maintain a healthy blood glucose level, or they are unable to produce insulin on their own. This unstable blood glucose can cause many serious conditions and is known to kill if left untreated.

According to a survey conducted in 2015, over 30 million Americans live with diabetes, which is over 90% of the population. This is serious, especially since it one of the leading causes of death in the country.

Chronic levels of high inflammation are known to lead to diabetes, as this inflammation is mostly what causes insulin resistance, which is what leads to type II diabetes. Oxidative stress of the cells may also play a role in the development of this disease. But, CBD is not only an antioxidant that will help prevent oxidative stress, but it is also highly anti-inflammatory. Studies have shown that people who regularly use CBD oil have lower levels of insulin and cholesterol. It may also help with other symptoms of diabetes such as weight, neuropathy, and retinopathy.

Scientists have discovered that there are a large number of cannabinoid receptors within the pancreas, which is likely the reason that CBD is known to have such an effect on this disease. Using CBD can trigger the pancreas and help it better understand how to process or make insulin.

Skin conditions and sensitivity are also common in diabetics, such as rashes, sores on the feet, burning, and itching. But, the natural healing properties of CBD paired with its anti-inflammatory and moisturizing benefits can greatly lessen various skin ailments. This is especially true when the CBD is applied topically as an oil, lotion, cream, lip balm, or salve.

Obesity

Obesity is a major problem, and it is only growing. With the abundance and ease of fast food and junk food spreading across the globe, more people are becoming overweight and obese. While there is nothing wrong with being fat or having curves, some people simply don't want this added weight. Being at a higher body fat percentage is also known to cause more diseases especially when it is abdominal fat. Yet, the rates of obesity are simply climbing especially in America.

According to a survey conducted in 2013, over 70% of adults are either overweight or obese. This survey revealed that over 17% of children and adolescences are either overweight or obese. We need to do better and promote a healthy body image while still promoting physical health.

While CBD is not a miracle cure, it will not make you

thin if you are eating a diet full of junk food; it is shown to help aid in weight loss. In a Korean study published in the Molecular and Cellular Biochemistry scientific journal, it was revealed that CBD could help with this weight loss in multiple ways.

Firstly, CBD has the ability to stimulate proteins and genes that increase the breakdown of body fat. It is also able to increase the number of mitochondria cells to increase the burning of calories and fat and decrease the amount of fat cells being produced.

When these three effects work together, it can turn our unhealthy white fat into healthy brown one. Unlike white fat, brown fat does not promote disease. It also has the ability to burn calories into energy. Animal studies show that this type of fat may also help prevent diabetes.

Sleep Disorders

CBD has been found to be able to increase sleep, which is especially important because 79% of Americans are sleep-deprived. To stay healthy, it is important to get between 7 to 8 hours of sleep every night. Yet, some people are still unable to get adequate sleep despite making time in their schedules for a healthy sleep routine. This is because over 50 million adults in America suffer from some type of sleep disorder. Insomnia is by far the most common, but thankfully, CBD has been shown to help with insomnia, regulation of the sleep cycle, deeper sleep, and prevent daytime sleepiness. Two common causes of insomnia are pain and anxiety, which CBD can also improve.

If you are at your wit's end because of your lack of sleep and you feel as if there are no options to help, then why not try CBD? Not only may it help your sleep disorder, but other symptoms and conditions that disrupt your life as well.

Cancer

Cancer is a deadly and dangerous disease, and it is only becoming more prevalent. Yet, there is hope, and you can keep up the fight. The anecdotal evidence of CBD, either from hemp or cannabis, is that it can heal cancer. Isn't it amazing? In fact, in many states where medical cannabis is legalized, you can use it for the management and treatment of cancer.

Not only does CBD actively prevent the growth of cancer cells, but it can also reduce the size of tumors. It is even more powerful when you take a full-spectrum form of CBD that contains the terpenes, as many of these terpenes have also been proven to have anti-cancer properties.

Along with helping treat cancer directly, CBD can also help reduce the symptoms of chemotherapy. It has the ability to reduce nausea and vomiting, decrease pain, stimulate the appetite, and reduce inflammation levels.

Epilepsy

Worldwide, an estimated 50 million people live with epilepsy, making it the most common type of neurological disease. This is a neurological condition which causes a person to have repeated seizures.

People with epilepsy frequently are unable to drive and have a difficult time maintaining a career, preparing food, or caring for children. These people can also be injured during their seizures. And, due to misinformation on how to help people who are having seizures, it can become a traumatic experience. These people are often held down and have wallets forced into their mouths, both of which are something you should never do to someone having a seizure.

Thankfully, the Food and Drug Administration in America has approved CBD as a treatment for epilepsy. This is especially wonderful, as there are many people who are resistant to drug therapy. While an average of two-thirds of epileptic patients can find a successful anticonvulsant medication on the first or second try, for a third of the cases, this is unsuccessful. This third of people are unlike to find any medicine that successfully prevents or reduces their seizures. This means that these people must rely on diets, surgeries, and natural medicine to treat their epilepsy.

Thankfully, CBD has a long history of being used to treat seizures, even in the most severe and rare cases. A study conducted in 2003, even found that CBD is able to provide benefits to epilepsy treatment that you are unable to find in prescription drugs.

One group of researchers has studied the effect of CBD and cannabis on epilepsy and other conditions for over 10 years now. This study proved that CBD can reduce seizure activity. They found that it can do this by activating the cannabinoid receptors in the brain and nervous system.

In animal studies, it has been found that CBD is more

effective in the treatment of epilepsy than THC. This means that even if you don't live in a state where you have access to medical cannabis, you can still make use of hemp CBD oil in your treatment.

Alzheimer's Disease

One of the leading causes of death and constantly on the rise, Alzheimer's disease is currently afflicting 5.7 million Americans. These numbers as suspected to rise to 14 million by the year 2050. This disease is devastating, but CBD has been shown to help treat both Alzheimer's and various forms of dementia.

In a study on CBD, it was found that it can reduce one of the causes of neuron damage in Alzheimer's disease. It was also able to help new healthy neurons grow and improve cognitive functioning.

One recent study on Alzheimer's and CBD found that not only the compound can decrease inflammation found in the brain, but it can also reduce damaging oxygen build up and the decline of brain cells.

Spinal Cord Injuries

There is an average of 17,700 spinal cord injuries each year in America, and those only include the people who survive long enough to make it to the hospital. These injuries are debilitating and can cause permanent disability.

However, CBD has been shown to be an excellent option for treating these injuries. Not only is CBD non-addictive and equally as effective as opioids, but it is also low in side effects. Even better, the CBD can directly help heal the injury and the various symptoms it causes. For instance, CBD has been proven to directly improve motor function and muscle plasticity. The reduction of inflammation and the neuron protection offered by this compound can also greatly benefit those with spinal cord injuries.

Attention Deficit Hyperactivity Disorder (ADHD)

Attention Deficit Hyperactivity Disorder is known by several names, including ADHD, ADD, hyperactivity, and hyperkinetic disorder in the U.K. This condition is highly under-diagnosed, especially in girls due to social sexism. However, in America at this time, an average of 11% of children are diagnosed with ADHD.

While many people assume ADHD only affects children, it will affect people of all ages and most children grow up with it to still struggle well into adulthood. This can be especially alienating for the children who never received a diagnosis and do not know why they are different from everyone else around them.

While there are many symptoms of ADHD, some of the classic symptoms include fidgeting, talking a lot, impulse control, difficulty in focusing, and an inability to stay on task. This may sound like a typical child behavior to some, but the degree that children experience these symptoms is much different from neurotypical children. This is especially evident in adults with ADHD.

While Ritalin, Adderall, and other drugs may help

control some peoples' ADHD, for others, it causes negative side effects and is ineffective. They have to search for a new treatment plan but do not know where to turn to.

Thankfully, CBD has been shown to help ADHD. In a study published in 2015, it was proven that cannabis could help adult patients with ADHD who are unable to take traditional drug therapy.

In another study, patients taking a CBD and THC compound greatly improved compared to a placebo group.

Addiction

Worldwide, people struggle with addiction and substance abuse. Even if you do not struggle with this, it is likely that someone you care about does. One study published in 2011, found that over 20 million Americans live with addiction. A shocking 100 people die every single day due to a drug overdose. This means that nearly 37,000 people die of a drug overdose a year. This is not even including those suffering from alcoholism.

Surprisingly, CBD may even aid in reducing addiction. A double-blind placebo study was conducted with those suffering from heroin addiction. In this study, it was found that a single dose of CBD daily greatly lessened cravings, unlike with the placebo group. Even after the study discontinued the use of CBD, the beneficial effects lasted for a week.

Another study found that people who were quitting smoking were able to reduce their urge to smoke by 40%

when using CBD administered through an inhaler. This is quite a large decrease, especially since the placebo group experienced no change in their urge to smoke.

While some people may worry about CBD being addicting, it is non-addictive and non-psychoactive. By increasing long-term synaptic plasticity, CBD can even help your brain "reprogram" itself so that it gradually begins to crave less of the addictive substance.

Parkinson's Disease

Parkinson's Disease is a common progressive nervous system disease which is only increasing in number. In fact, statistics show that by 2020 nearly a million people within America will be living with Parkinson's. This disease is known for affecting movement and it does this with tremors, difficulty walking or moving, and partial paralysis.

Although, since this is a nervous system disease, that means CBD has a great ability to help manage and treat it. Since the endocannabinoid system is able to regulate the lifespan of cells, it can protect and heal brain cells, as well as replacing damaged ones. A double-blind study published in 2014 found that treating those with Parkinson's disease with CBD is effective and leads to a significant improvement in both symptoms and quality of life in the participants.

Fibromyalgia

Fibromyalgia affects an estimated 10 million people within America, and it is known to cause full-body pain, deep muscular pain, fatigue, insomnia, migraines, dizziness, cognitive difficulties, irritable bowel syndrome, and allergies. Though not all of these symptoms have to be present for a person to have fibromyalgia, they can vary from person to person.

While fibromyalgia does not usually reveal high inflammation on typical blood tests and is resistant to anti-inflammatory drugs, it has now been revealed that it may have an inflammation component after all. A study published in the Journal of Pain and Research during 2017 was able to find inflammation in fibromyalgia patients after more extensive testing. After exploring nearly 100 types of inflammation, the researchers were able to find extensive systemic inflammation as well as central nervous system inflammation.

A study by Dr. Genevra Liptan found that the layer of connective tissue wrapped around and protecting the brain is often inflamed in patients with fibromyalgia. Dr. Liptan surmises that this inflammation around the brain is what causes the frequent pain and other symptoms that people with fibromyalgia experience.

Not only is CBD able to help pain from a variety of sources, but it could help reduce the inflammation prominent in people with fibromyalgia. Therefore, it wouldn't just treat the pain, but also the cause of the pain.

In a survey conducted by the National Pain Foundation, after interviewing over 1,300 people, it was found that medical cannabis is more effective in treating fibromyalgia pain than the current prescriptions on the market. While many people try medication after medication for fibromyalgia to only find little relief and many side effects, 62% of the patients on cannabis found improvement. This is a much higher rate of success than with traditional drug therapy, and with the ability to potentially manage the root cause of fibromyalgia, it is an exciting prospect.

Multiple Sclerosis

Multiple sclerosis is a progressive degenerative disease that affects the central nervous system. This devastating condition is currently affecting approximately 400,000 people in America, and 10,000 new cases are diagnosed every year.

This condition is caused when the immune system begins to attack and degrade the protection of our nerve fibers, which prevents the brain from being able to communicate with our body. Eventually, this condition causes the nerves to become permanently damaged. Symptoms and severity vary from person to person, and it is well-known that lifestyle factors affect multiple sclerosis.

In a European-Canadian study, it was found that a combination of CBD and THC together can greatly improve muscle plasticity, muscle spasms, neuropathic pain, and sleep in patients with multiple sclerosis. In another study, cannabis extract was compared against placebo for a 12-week period. During this time, it was found that the muscle stiffness in the cannabis group improved by two-fold.

Multiple sclerosis is well-known to not only cause inflammation, but much of its damage is caused by this very same inflammation. However, the properties of CBD are naturally anti-inflammatory.

Nausea and Vomiting

Nausea and vomiting can be symptoms of a wide array of illnesses and disease. People with gastrointestinal disorders, cancer, nervous system disorders, anxiety, and more often experience these symptoms. While some people may figure that nausea isn't too bad if you are unable to eat adequate food, it can become highly detrimental, further affecting your health. Not only that, but it greatly interferes with peoples' social and professional lives. Simply taking a sip of a drink or eating a single bite of food could send someone to the bathroom, unable to contain the contents of their stomach. Even if they can manage to get the food down, the nausea is so severe that they cannot concentrate on anything else and they never know when they will vomit.

However, multiple studies have shown that both CBD and THC can help alleviate these symptoms. Whether you are using THC-free CBD oil or cannabis, which contains both CBD and THC, both of these compounds are shown to help. In fact, cannabis has been used to treat these various symptoms for centuries in ancient medicine.

The British Journal of Pharmacology published a paper which found that CBD is able to alleviate the symptoms of nausea and vomiting by triggering the serotonin receptor. The serotonin released by this receptor communicates with the vomiting center in the brain to help calm things down. It can also help create a natural enzyme to increase appetite and improve digestion.

Asthma and Chronic Obstructive Pulmonary Disease

Both asthma and chronic obstructive pulmonary disease, otherwise known as COPD, are characterized by chronic inflammation in the lungs. This is a common problem, as 26.5 million Americans live with asthma and an average of 16 million live with COPD. Yet, it is estimated that millions more live with COPD and simply haven't been diagnosed.

Every year in America, 1.3 million visits to the emergency room is a result of asthma, which is the most common childhood illness. Every year this condition causes 3,500 deaths. Over 3 million people die a year due to COPD.

But, an answer may lie in hemp and cannabis. For thousands of years, these plants have been used to treat a variety of lung disorders. CBD is able to help by activating the CB2 receptors, which reduce the inflammation in the lungs and acts as a bronchodilator. THC is helpful as well, as it also acts as a bronchodilator by activating the CB1 receptors on the bronchial nerve endings.

People who have asthma tend to have hyperreactive airways that contract when they shouldn't. This can cause the airways to become obstructed and results in troubled breathing. However, a German study published in the Institute for Clinical Pharmacology found that an endocannabinoid neurotransmitter may be able to prevent this obstruction. This neurotransmitter is known as anandamide.

When someone's airways are triggered and begin to contract, anandamide increases to combat the reaction. The higher the amount of anandamide the milder the reaction. As on example, someone who had a slightly mild reaction had high levels of anandamide.

CBD is able to increase this endocannabinoid neurotransmitter by preventing an enzyme from breaking down the anandamide. By preventing it from breaking down, the levels of anandamide can increase to combat the asthmatic reaction.

Mucus is another asthma of lung conditions which causes obstruction of the airways, coughing, and difficulty breathing. The cytokine (small proteins) IL-13 are largely the cause of this mucus increase. CBD has been found to decrease the amount of this protein, which allows people with lung conditions to breathe easier and better expel the mucus from their lungs.

Migraines

Migraines may seem to some people as "just a little headache", but its sufferers know that there is nothing "little" about a migraine. The pain is so severe that people can lose their vision and become unable to handle sound, light, walking, eating, and more. This condition is the sixth leading cause of disability and 39 million people in America suffer from them. Of these people, an average of 4 million has migraines every single day.

Thankfully, CBD oil can offer relief. This compound is able to relieve pain, vomiting, nausea, light sensitivity, and much more. A 2016 study found that people who began medical cannabis reduced from having seizures ten times a month to only four times.

Another study in 2010, found that the endocannabinoid system is connected to migraines and that activating this system through CBD could be a beneficial treatment option for people with chronic migraines.

As you can see, there are many health benefits to using CBD oil. The benefits listed in this chapter, and many others, have been studied and regularly show beneficial results.

Chapter 3: How to Choose and Buy CBD Oil

The industry for medicinal hemp and cannabis is on the rise. With scientific knowledge of the various therapeutic properties growing and proving that it's a safe option, more laws are becoming loosening both internationally and at the state level. Because of this, the industry to produce cannabis, hemp, and CBD oil is booming. The industry is growing so quickly that it will soon be worth $13 billion in America alone. A large number of choices to get the exact product you need is great, but it can also leave people confused and uncertain about which product is right for them.

You may be able to find CBD oil both online and in retail stores, but you want to be sure that the oil you are finding is of high quality and pure. You don't want to buy some snake oil that will deteriorate your health rather than improve it. Thankfully, if you know what to look for, you can find a high-quality CBD oil with all of the therapeutic qualities you require. In this chapter, you will learn about how to find the right brand for you and even a list of some of the most renowned brands.

Most of us have to factor cost into our decision, but we still need to ensure the product we buy is of decent quality. You may find that some bottles are more expensive, but they might actually be a better deal than the cheaper bottles in the long run. This is because, oftentimes, brands will have more expensive bottles of CBD that are a higher concentration. This means that the dose is smaller in actuality and you won't go through a single bottle as quickly. For instance, a single 500 mg bottle might cost less than two 250 mg bottles. To determine which bottle is the best value, calculate how many doses each bottle provides against the price.

It is important to decide whether you want CBD isolates or full-spectrum. The isolates, also known as crystals, are pure CBD that has been refined. Some people prefer these for baking due to their lack of flavor. Or, they may simply dislike the flavor of hemp and cannabis.

Although, in general, it is often best to purchase full-spectrum instead, if you can. These are CBD oils that still contain the valuable terpenes and if you don't have the terpenes, you will be missing out on many health benefits.

You need to decide what concentration of CBD you require for where you are at and your symptoms. Some people may be able to manage their symptoms with a relatively small concentration of CBD, otherwise known as dose size. Yet, some people may have a more difficult case and require a larger dose. Either way, you shouldn't start out at the highest concentration.

Think about it this way: doctors often start people on a small dose of medication before they bump them up and find their therapeutic dose. This therapeutic dose is the amount the person needs to control their symptoms and varies from person to person.

You don't want to start out on the highest dose, so start at a low to moderate dose and you can gradually increase this over the period of few days or weeks until you begin to attain your desired results.

There are many delivery methods you can try for CBD. It is important to either pick which method you prefer or try a few methods and find what you like. Some of the most popular delivery methods are dropper bottles for sublingual ingestion and baking, capsules, vaporizers, and crystals.

The dropper bottles are ideal because the sublingual delivery, meaning placing the drop directly under your tongue, is effective. By ingesting the oil, it will benefit your entire body. And, when placed under the tongue rather than on top of your tongue, it is more quickly able to be absorbed and utilized by your body.

Capsules are helpful when you want an accessible and convenient option for on-the-go. Like the dropper method, these are ingested so that they help your entire system. Though, they take longer to be digested and used by your body than the sublingual method. This method is also preferred by some people because it doesn't have a taste.

When using a vaporizer or crystals, it is important to look at the ingredients list because they often have added ingredients and you want to know exactly what you are consuming.

Some people also prefer topical treatments such as balms, lotions, bath salts, salves, and even lip balms. These are helpful because while it may not be as powerful of an effect as directly ingesting the CBD, you can place it where you are in pain. So, if you injured a knee or wrist, then you can place the CBD skin product directly on your joint to experience relief.

Choosing the extraction method of the CBD you are purchasing is extremely important. Some cheaper brands may cut corners and use toxic and harmful solvents to remove the CBD from the plant. These include ingredients such as propane, butane, pentane, and hexane. These ingredients are often with gas stoves and ranges, and some of the chemicals eventually end up in the finished product.

The highest quality CBD products are usually made with the supercritical CO_2 extraction method. With this method, a large machine is able to use carbon dioxide that is at supercritical high pressure. This enables it to isolate the CBD from the plant, separate it, and maintain its purity. With this method, they can either keep the terpenes or remove them completely. While this process is more expensive, it creates a high-quality pure product without the use of toxic substances.

While a little less pure than the CO_2, the ethanol extraction is less expensive and still high-quality. This method uses non-toxic food-grade alcohol which also retains the terpenes, which is good for added health benefits.

Finally, CBD can also be extracted into oil, such as olive oil or coconut oil. This type of extraction method is not as potent, but it contains the terpenes and isn't as expensive. While the supercritical CO_2 extraction method may be ideal, if you are on a budget and can't afford ethanol extracted CBD, then you may need to settle for oil extraction.

Any reputable manufacturer will be open and transparent about how they extract their products. If they are not open about this, then you will want to be extremely cautious. I recommend against using any company that is not open and honest.

Choose where your CBD is derived from. While both cannabis

and hemp originate from the cannabis sativa genus, they have different characteristics by being selectively bred over the centuries. For instance, cannabis-derived CBD is illegal in most of the states across America due to its THC content. On the other hand, hemp-derived CBD is regularly tested to ensure that it does not contain over a certain percentage of THC. Because of this, hemp-derived CBD oil is legal in most of the States.

But, choosing where your CBD is derived from entails more than choose cannabis or hemp. You also need to choose where it was grown and under what conditions.

There are some trusted European brands that have been operating longer than CBD has been legal in America. These brands undergo strict European regulation. However, there are some trusted American brands as well. When choosing where your CBD is derived from, whether Europe or America, try to find a brand that is certified organic.

Be sure that you know exactly where it is grown. If the company doesn't specify whether it was grown in Europe or America, then it is likely that it is industrialized hemp that was grown somewhere overseas. These plants are often grown in places with little environmental regulations. This is dangerous, as hemp and cannabis plants are bio-accumulators, which means that the plant will absorb any toxins and heavy metals from the soil and air around them. It is imperative that the plant is grown in a healthy environment.

Many people who are desperate and on a budget may not look too far into a brand when purchasing CBD. They may simply buy some off of Amazon or a page that pulled up on Google, without looking in-depth into the brand and their practices. It is important that you know all about the brand you are purchasing from, and because the U.S Food and Drug Administration has found that some places that sell "CBD oil" are in actuality selling little more than snake oil.

So, how do you know if the CBD oil you are buying is legit? It should be tested by a third-party laboratory. Reputable brands will have their products regularly tested and they provide their results on the website. If you can't find the results on their website, but they mention having them, you can always contact their customer service and request a copy of the results.

These lab results will reveal the potency of CBD, whether or not it has THC, other cannabinoids within the product, terpenes, pesticides, heavy metals, and other dangerous contaminants. If you want to ensure your product is high-quality and safe, there is no better way than with a third-party laboratory result. I recommend against buying from any brand that doesn't have these available.

Following is a list of some popular brands. But, remember, a brand may change over time. What once was a reputable brand may begin to use lower standards or come under new management. For this reason, please always check the company's website, look to see where the CBD was grown, how it was extracted, and if they have any recent third-party laboratory results.

Charlotte's Web

One of the original CBD products on the American

market, Charlotte's Web was started by the same Stanley Brothers who helped Charlotte Figi. We previously mentioned Charlotte and how the Stanley Brothers helped her parents get a high-quality CBD oil to help control her Dravet's syndrome.

After the success with Charlotte, the Stanley Brothers not only named the strain of hemp after her but also their brand. Once they saw how much it was able to help young Charlotte, they decided to make the strain available to other people as well. This strain is now available in most States and can be found on their website.

The Charlotte's Web products are free of pesticides and GMOs. They are also in the process of being certified organic and certified as having a Good Manufacturing Practice. Their facility is also registered with the FDA.

Charlotte's Web has a variety of products, including CBD oils with or without flavorings, capsules, balm, cream, and even oil for pets.

Bluebird Botanicals

Bluebird Botanicals is grown and processed in Colorado before being shipped across the nation. Their extraction methods are safe; their main process is by using ethanol and also using supercritical CO_2 on some of their products. Their products are tested by third-party laboratories regularly and they make these results easy to find on their product's page. They offer a variety of price points, but overall they are reasonably priced.

Bluebird Botanicals offers extracts of their oils, as well

as concentrated extracts, capsules, isolates, and vaping products.

Some of their products have added benefits, such as the Complete Blend. This blend contains hemp that has been raw and heated and has different health benefits. It also contains terpenes; their Signature Blend contains added black seed oil and frankincense; they have a vape oil which you can simply add to a vape pen; and, they have capsules that you can give to your pets who may be ill or if you simply want to increase their health and quality of life.

Theramu

Different from most brands, Theramu uses emu oil as a carrier oil for their products. This is because they claim that emu oil is a near-perfect carrier for CBD, enabling the CBD to be absorbed more quickly and effectively. Their products are free of THC and tested by a third-party laboratory.

Theramu has a range of unique products not offered elsewhere, including soothing bath crystals made with Epsom salt, CBD isolate, emu oil, eucalyptus, lavender, and camphor, both in regular and extra concentrated strengths; pain relieving balm with CBD isolate, emu oil, beeswax, eucalyptus, and camphor; mango-flavored sublingual "elixir" extract; beard grooming balm with CBD and essential oils; and, moisturizing under-eye serum containing CBD isolate and emu oil.

BioCBD Plus

BioCBD Plus is different than most because their products are water-soluble. This enables them to be better absorbed by our bodies. This is because we are only able to absorb a certain percentage of fat-soluble CBD since our bodies are made up of mostly water. Because of this, BioCBD Plus promises that you will be getting the full benefit of what you pay for when you buy from them.

Another great aspect of their company is that every time you buy a bottle of the CBD, they will donate a bottle into a program where they will give out CBD products to chronically ill and disabled people who are unable to afford it themselves.

BioCBD Plus grows their hemp in Scandinavia. It is organic, GMO-free, and they don't add any artificial colors, sugar, or artificial flavorings. You can easily find their lab tests on their website.

Their products include capsules, muscle and joint pain relief oil, and vape cartridges.

Elixinol

Elixinol is well-renowned, high-quality, and multiple award-winning CBD company from Europe. Their products are organic, GMO-free, utilized through the supercritical CO_2 extraction method, still contain the terpenes, and they are third-party tested by an independent laboratory. Not only are their products third-party tested, but Elixinol will even send out tainted test samples along with the accurate samples on purpose. The purpose of this is to look at both results and see if the laboratory is being honest and accurate.

Elixinol's product line includes tinctures, capsules, liposomes, vacuum-sealed pen, and dog treats.

Their liposome line differentiates itself from other brands as it is created in a way to be easily, quickly, and effectively absorbed by the body. This works because liposomes are small spheres of cholesterol and phospholipids, which can be absorbed by both water and fat. This enabled the body to absorb it better.

Entourage Hemp

Entourage Hemp uses a 'WholeFlower' Principle. This principle believes that while the stems, stalks, and roots of the hemp flower have some therapeutic properties, nearly all of the benefits originate from the seeds, trichomes, and tissues naturally found in the flower of the hemp. Therefore, they work to use this more potent and effective part of the hemp plant.

Entourage Hemp also grows their hemp on organic farms in Colorado, practices the Good Manufacturing Practices rules established by the FDA, uses the supercritical CO_2 extraction method along with the ethanol extraction method, have their products tested by third-party laboratories, and their entire e-liquid like is Kosher.

Entourage Hemp has three main products, which include tinctures, soft-gels, and e-liquids for vaping.

Receptra Naturals

Receptra Naturals is a brand grown on a family farm in the state of Colorado. All of their products are extracted with ethanol from the flower of the plant, fully organic, and third-party tested.

Receptra Naturals has a few different lines of products, including Health and Wellness Extracts, Active Lifestyle Extracts, Topicals, Receptra Lip Balm, and Receptra Pet. Their extracts are flavored, which is ideal for people who don't care for the flavor of hemp and children.

Vape Bright

Vape Bright is wonderful because unlike some vaping brands, they truly value having high-quality and pure CBD without any added toxins. All of their products are made with high-quality and organic hemp, which are then tested by a third-party laboratory. The test results of their products are easy to find and read.

Unlike most vaping brands, they keep the health-promoting beneficial terpenes. Vape Bright also refrains from adding fillers such as vegetable glycerin or propylene glycol, which other brands frequently use.

You can purchase rechargeable vape cartridges, battery packs, and starter kits from Vape Bright.

While there may be some snake oil brands out there falsely claiming to sell "CBD", if you know how to pick out a good brand that fits your needs, then you will be in good hands. The well-respected brands that run third-party testing are not only safe, but they are also high-quality.

Chapter 4: How to Dose and Safely Consume CBD Oil

There is often a confusion on how to get the correct dose of CBD and what form to choose. In this chapter, we will explore how to find your correct dosage, the best ways to consume CBD, and even how to safely give CBD products to your pets.

Some people may wonder if certain conditions need specific blends or dosage sizes. At this point, there is no clinical evidence to support that some conditions may need different blends. Though, some may need different dosages.

For instance, if you live where cannabis is legalized, then you could purchase a blend that is one part THC to one part CBD, or two parts CBD to one part THC. This could work great for you but may have a little effect on someone else. This is because finding your exact needs take a little trial and error. For this reason, medical dispensaries will often give people a couple of different blends to try out. This enables the person to find what their body best responds to.

Even if you find a perfect blend for you, this may change over time. While it may be frustrating when your body's needs change, it's because our natural physiology changes over time. This physiological change includes our endocannabinoid system, their receptors, and how they respond to stimuli. This may mean that over time, you will occasionally need to tinker with your dosage or your blend.

While it would be lovely if there was a one-size-fits-all dosage of CBD, this is simply not how our bodies react to medication, whether that medication is pharmaceutical or natural. There is a study on mice which illustrates this nicely.

In the study, the researchers were testing multiple mice all on the same dosage of THC. Yet, the mice reacted differently. Despite having the same dosage, they experienced different cellular effects and exhibited different behaviors. In this study, the changes tended to vary based on the age of the mice.

This is extremely common in medicine, and this is why many doctors begin their patients on a small dose of medication before increasing the dose over time. Medications, including the natural ones, can bind to different receptors depending on the dosage. While it's not always the case, generally, somewhere around a mid-sized dose works for most people.

You may think that doubling the dose will also double the benefits, but that is not necessarily true. In fact, sometimes, doubling the dose will decrease the number of benefits. This is likely because when you are consuming a low dose of CBD, it can only affect a certain number of receptors. Therefore, it naturally targets the receptors that it has the most affinity with and will make the most impact. But, if the dose is greatly increased, then the receptors may become overly saturated.

However, some people may benefit from a higher dose. While people with illnesses such as anxiety often find the most benefit from a moderate dose, studies have found that higher doses can be effective for some illnesses or disorders, especially epilepsy.

Clinical trials treating epilepsy with CBD have been able to utilize increasingly high doses, without the CBD becoming less effective or changing the way in which the participants responded. Some of these trials are giving the epileptic patients hundreds of milligrams of CBD every day. It is worth mentioning, though, that these are CBD capsules. This is important because when taken as a capsule, CBD isn't bioavailable; therefore, only a fraction of it can be absorbed by the bloodstream.

Speaking of the form in which you administer your CBD, we have already mentioned the various benefits of sublingual oil, capsules, and topical ointments, but, what about vaping?

Whether or not you are someone who already vapes, you might want to give CBD vaping a try. This is because vaping allows your body to quickly and effectively absorb the benefits. While edibles and sublingual CBD consumption may have its benefits, they do not offer the immediate relief that comes with vaping. This is because when you vape CBD, it can reach your bloodstream by going through your lungs, rather than being required to go through the long digestion process. This allows people to feel relief within either a few seconds to a few minutes. If you are someone who is suffering from anxiety attacks, pain, or anything else where you need immediate relief, then you might appreciate vaping.

There is also evidence that CBD could possibly be more bioavailable when vaped than when consumed in edibles. One study conducted on the bioavailability of THC found that when baked in cookies, it was only 6% bioavailable. Whereas, when the THC was inhaled, it was 18% bioavailable. This study should be taken with a grain of salt since THC and CBD are slightly different. But, these two compounds are also similarly absorbed by the body, so this study sheds some light on how CBD might be absorbed by our bodies.

Another benefit of vaping is that when you buy edibles like gummies or choose capsules, then you are unable to completely customize your dosage. On the other hand, when you vape you can decide the exact amount of vape oil you wish to add. This way you can adjust your dose down to the drop for what you feel is best for your body.

If you are someone who feels hesitant to take a pill, oil, or ointment out in public, then you might also prefer vaping, especially if you are someone who already vapes. Most people will assume you are vaping an e-cigarette and won't know that it is CBD. This can be beneficial for people who feel insecure about CBD or are worried about it being stigmatized.

If you are trying to determine which method of CBD to try first, I most recommend sublingual drops and vaping. Edibles are a wonderful way to work it into your daily life and diet. Ointments, lotions, and other topical applications are helpful if you want to put the CBD on a specific injury or painful location. And, I would least recommend capsules, unless they are a brand specifically designed for increased bioavailability.

If you are looking to consume your CBD in edibles, there are a couple of things to keep in mind when cooking or baking.

Firstly, CBD is fat-soluble. This not only affects how well it absorbs in our bodies, but it also affects cooking. Unless you buy a water-soluble brand of CBD, then you will need to put it in additional fat while baking. It doesn't matter whether the fat is olive oil, coconut oil, butter, or shortening. You can use your preference, but make sure that it is fully combined into the fat source before you add it to your recipe.

However, there is an exception. Some alcohols can support CBD. These include alcohols such as rum, vodka, and whiskey. Water-based alcohols, such as beer and wine, are unable to carry the CBD and should be avoided.

Secondly, you need to be incredibly mindful of the importance of the temperature when you cook or bake it. While heat may help CBD absorb more effectively into your system, it can also cook away some of the benefits if the temperature is too hot.

CBD will begin to evaporate at above 350° Fahrenheit, so you always want to keep the heat below that. Be sure not to place the CBD on direct heat either, as it will also cause some of the CBD to evaporate.

You have heard all about CBD for yourself, but what about for your furry friend? Just like humans, animals have endocannabinoid systems as well. This means that CBD products can also help your little friend. In fact, more and more people are now giving their pets CBD products to either treat illness or as a preventative.

If you have a cat or a dog that suffers from anxiety, chronic pain, asthma, or some other conditions, you may want to discuss CBD with your veterinarian. While many studies have shown CBD to be safe, there are some important aspects you should keep in mind.

First, if your pet is in hepatic medication, then they should avoid CBD as it can block the absorption just as grapefruit does in humans. Some pets may experience side effects, though at the correct dosage this is rare. These side effects are usually drowsiness or dry mouth.

Due to the small size of pets, some people might give them the wrong dose. To determine the dosage your pet requires, simply follow the directions from the manufacturer according to their species and size. This will vary, although the dosage is usually only a few drops 2 or 3 times daily.

You can get CBD products in various forms for pets, including in drops, tablets, and treats. More brands are beginning to release their own pet-specific CBD lines, such as Bluebird Botanicals. There are also brands specifically for your furry friend, such as Pet Releaf, Canna-Pets, and Innovet.

Whether you need a small dose or a large dose, edibles or vaping, or wish to use CBD on yourself or your furry friend, there are many options when it comes to CBD. When figuring out your dose, take your time and work slowly to find what works best for you.

Chapter 5: Cooking with CBD Oil

In this chapter, you will be provided with all the recipes you need to enjoy baked goods complimented with CBD. Whether you want sweets or something savory, there is something here for everyone. The CBD oil in these recipes can be altered depending on your taste and the strength of CBD oil you have. You can also use pure CBD oil complete with the terpenes for the most benefit, or you can use CBD isolate if you prefer not to taste the CBD within your finished product.

If you are new to baking with CBD, you may want to use only half of the oil called for in these recipes until you get used to the flavor. If you are trying a recipe for the first time, then consider only making half of a batch so that if you dislike it, you don't waste the ingredients.

Above all else, remember that cooking with CBD has many health benefits, can be incredibly tasty, and especially fun!

Carrot Zucchini Muffins

These muffins are healthy, sweet, and moist. The addition of the grated fruits and vegetables not only prevents them from being dry, but it greatly increases the flavor as well. While the pecans add a heavenly crunch, you can replace them with another nut or omit them completely depending on your preference.

Servings: 12
Prep time: 10 minutes
Cooking time: 20 minutes

Calories: 235 kcal
Fat: 12g
Protein: 2g
Carbs: 26g
Net Carbs: 25g

Ingredients:

- Zucchini, grated – .5 cup

- Apple, grated – .5 cup

- Carrot, grated – .5 cup

- All-purpose flour – 1.5 cups

- Eggs – 1

- White sugar – .75 cup

- Light olive oil – .5 cup

- CBD oil – 1 tablespoon

- Cinnamon – .5 teaspoon

- Baking soda – .5 teaspoon

- Sea salt – .5 teaspoon

- Pecans, chopped – .5 cup (optional)

Instructions:

1. In a medium-sized mixing bowl, combine the light olive oil and CBD oil. Then, add in the eggs and white sugar.
2. In another bowl, combine the all-purpose flour, cinnamon, baking soda, and sea salt. Then, add in the flour mixture into the wet mixture.

3. Gently fold the grated zucchini, apple, and carrot along with the chopped pecans into the muffin batter.

4. Scoop the muffin batter evenly into 12 lined muffin cups and bake until they are fully done all the way through. This should take about 20 to 25 minutes at 350° F. You will know the muffins are ready when a toothpick is inserted and removed from the center of the muffins and it remains clean.

Pumpkin Spice Muffins

Whether it is autumn or spring, these muffins are perfect for either breakfast, snack, or dessert. These muffins are moist and have a perfect balance of pumpkin and spices.

Servings: 12
Prep time: 6 minutes
Cooking time: 20 minutes

Calories: 261 kcal
Fat: 15.6g
Protein: 4.7g
Carbs: 29.6g
Net Carbs: 25.8g

Ingredients:

- Dark brown sugar – .5 cup

- All-purpose flour – 1.5 cups

- Pumpkin puree – 15 ounces

- Eggs – 2

- Light olive oil – .5 cup

- CBD oil – 1 tablespoon

- Cloves, ground – .25 teaspoon

- Vanilla extract – 1 teaspoon

- White sugar – 1 cup

- Cinnamon – 2 teaspoons

- Sea salt – .5 teaspoon

- Nutmeg, ground – .25 teaspoon

- Baking soda – 1 teaspoon

Instructions:

1. In a large metal mixing bowl, combine the dark brown sugar, pumpkin puree, eggs, light olive oil, CBD oil, vanilla extract, and white sugar.
2. In a small mixing bowl, combine the all-purpose flour, cloves, cinnamon, sea salt, nutmeg, and baking soda. Gently fold into the wet mixture.
3. Divide the pumpkin muffin batter between 12 paper muffin liners, then bake in a preheated oven at 350° F.
4. The muffins are ready when a toothpick inserted in the center is removed clean, about 20 minutes. Enjoy!

Classic Bran Muffins

These muffins are delicious! They are perfect for when you want something healthy that is still a treat. The high-fiber content not only is better for your health but will also keep you full throughout your morning. Enjoy these as is or with your favorite nuts or fruits.

Servings: 6

Prep time: 10 minutes

Cooking time: 20 minutes

Calories: 276 kcal
Fat: 15.6g
Protein: 4.7g
Carbs: 29.6g
Net Carbs: 25.8g

Ingredients:

- Wheat bran – .5 cup

- Whole-wheat flour – .75 cup

- Greek yogurt – .25 cup

- White sugar – .33 cup

- All-purpose flour – .5 cup

- Eggs – 1

- Boiling water – .5 cup

- Olive oil – .33 cup

- Sea salt – .5 teaspoon

- Cinnamon – 2 teaspoons

- CBD oil – 1 tablespoon

- Baking powder – 1.5 teaspoons

- Nutmeg – .12 teaspoon

Instructions:

1. In a medium bowl, combine the boiling water with the wheat bran. Allow it to sit for 5 minutes before adding in the greek yogurt and the egg.
2. In another bowl, combine the whole-wheat flour, white sugar, all-purpose flour, sea salt, cinnamon, baking powder, and nutmeg. Then, add in the bran mixture.
3. In a measuring cup, combine the light olive oil and CBD oil, and then add it to the muffin batter.
4. Divide the bran muffin batter between 6 lined muffin cups and bake them until they are fully cooked. They should be firm, and a toothpick once inserted should come out clean. In an oven preheated at 350° F, it should take about 20 minutes.

Asparagus Gruyère Frittata

This Asparagus Gruyere Frittata is full of vegetables and cheese. This flavorful and healthy breakfast option is full of fiber and protein, helping to keep you healthy, strong, energized, and satisfied.

Servings: 4
Prep time: 15 minutes
Cooking time: 25 minutes

Calories: 286 kcal
Fat: 22.5g
Protein: 16.4g
Carbs: 3.6g
Net Carbs: 2.5g

Ingredients:

- Eggs, large – 8
- Olive oil – 2 tablespoons
- CBD oil – 1 tablespoon
- Sea salt – .5 teaspoon
- Water – 1 tablespoon
- Onion, diced – .5 cup
- Mushrooms, sliced – 1 cup
- Asparagus, chopped into one-inch slices – 1 cup
- Red bell pepper, diced – .5 cup
- Gruyère cheese, grated – .25 cup
- Black pepper, ground – to taste

Instructions:

1. In a medium bowl, whisk together the water, eggs, sea salt, and ground black pepper.
2. In a large 10" to 12" skillet, saute the diced onion over medium heat until translucent. Then, add in the sliced mushrooms and cook until they are tender. Stir in the sliced asparagus and cook until it is also tender. Lastly, add in the bell pepper until slightly softened.
3. Stir the CBD oil into the vegetables and then pour the egg mixture over the top. Use a spatula to move the eggs around so that they can cook all around the vegetables.
4. Once the vegetable frittata appears halfway set, sprinkle the grated Gruyère over the top and place it in the oven until it is done, about 12 to 15 minutes at 350° F.

5. Allow the frittata to cool for a few minutes before cutting and enjoy!

Vegan Fruit Snacks

These delicious fruit snacks will make you feel as if you are back in childhood. While the strawberry-kiwi mixture is delicious, feel free to mix it up and use your favorite fruits. Whether you are young or old, these snacks are the perfect way in which to enjoy your daily CBD.

Servings: 4
Prep time: 7 minutes
Cooking time: 10 minutes

Calories: 286 kcal
Fat: 10.3g
Protein: 0.7g
Carbs: 18g
Net Carbs: 17g

Ingredients:

- Strawberries, diced – 1 cup

- Kiwi, diced – 1 cup

- Water – .33 cup

- Honey – 2 tablespoons

- Coconut oil, melted – 2 tablespoons

- CBD oil – 1 tablespoon

- Agar powder – 4 teaspoons

Instructions:

1. In a blender, combine the strawberries, kiwi, water, and honey until it is completely smooth with no chunks remaining.
2. Add the fruit mixture and the agar powder into a medium-sized pot over medium heat. Bring it to a simmer, and then continue cooking it for 30 seconds before removing it from the heat.
3. In a small bowl, stir together the coconut oil and CBD oil, and then fully whisk it into the fruit mixture.
4. Spoon the strawberry kiwi mixture into small silicone molds. Allow it to set up in the fridge until firm, about 30 minutes.
5. Remove the fruit snacks from the molds and store in the fridge. Enjoy!

No-Bake Energy Bars

These energy bars are quick and easy, perfect for pre or post workout, on-the-go, or whenever you need a go-to snack. These flavorful bars combine coconut, honey, peanuts, and chocolate for an absolutely unbeatable flavor. If you have a peanut allergy, you can always replace the peanut butter with almond butter or sunflower seed butter.

Servings: 8
Prep time: 7 minutes
Cooking time: 0 minutes

Calories: 236 kcal
Fat: 15.7g
Protein: 3.5g

Carbs: 23.5g
Net Carbs: 21g

Ingredients:

- Quick-cooking oats – 1 cup
- Shredded coconut, unsweetened – 1 cup
- Creamy peanut butter – .5 cup
- CBD oil – 2 tablespoons
- Mini chocolate chips – .33 cup
- Honey – .33 cup
- Sea salt – .5 teaspoon
- Vanilla – .5 teaspoon

Instructions:

1. Combine the quick-cooking oats, shredded unsweetened coconut, and mini chocolate chips in a medium-sized mixing bowl.
2. In a small bowl, combine the creamy peanut butter and CBD oil. Then, add in the sea salt, vanilla, and honey. Stir to combine.
3. Add the wet ingredients to the oatmeal bowl and combine. If the mixture is too dry, add some extra honey. If it is too wet, add extra oats.
4. Place the energy bar mixture on a parchment lined 9" x 13" pan. Flatten it out evenly using a spatula. Cut the bars, and then place them in the refrigerator for an hour until the bars are solidified. Enjoy!

Home-Style Baked Fries

These delicious baked fries are complemented with the earthy rosemary, spicy garlic, and CBD oil. They are full of flavor on their own, but also taste amazing with any of your favorite dipping sauces.

Servings: 2
Prep time: 5 minutes
Cooking time: 20 minutes

Calories: 451 kcal
Fat: 18g
Protein: 8g
Carbs: 66.6g
Net Carbs: 61.7g

Ingredients:

- Russet potatoes, peeled – 2

- Olive oil – 2 tablespoons

- Sea salt – 1 teaspoon

- CBD oil – 2 teaspoons

- Garlic powder – .5 teaspoon

- Rosemary, dried – 1 teaspoon

Instructions:

1. Cut the potatoes into half-inch thick slices and place them on a baking sheet covered with a parchment paper.

2. Toss the potato slices in olive oil, sea salt, CBD oil, garlic powder, and rosemary.

3. Bake the fries at 350° F for about 15 to 20 minutes, until fully cooked through and crispy. Enjoy with your favorite dipping sauce!

Roasted Red Pepper Hummus

Whether you love hummus with fresh vegetables, in a wrap, or with your favorite Indian food, this roasted red pepper hummus will compliment a wide variety of dishes. The roasted red peppers compliment perfectly with the robust CBD and the peppery fresh garlic.

Servings: 6
Prep time: 10 minutes
Cooking time: 0 minutes

Calories: 235 kcal
Fat: 12.7g
Protein: 4g
Carbs: 11.7g
Net Carbs: 8.4g

Ingredients:

- Chickpeas, cooked – 15 ounces (equivalent to 1 can)

- Roasted red bell peppers, chopped and from a jar – .75 ounces

- Olive oil – 2 tablespoons

- CBD oil – 1.5 tablespoons

- Tahini – .25 cup

- Lemon juice – .25 cup

- Garlic, minced – 2 cloves

- Cumin, ground – .5 teaspoon

- Sea salt – to taste

Instructions:

1. In a food processor, combine the lemon juice and tahini until it becomes creamy, about a minute and a half. Halfway through, scrape down the sides.
2. Add in the olive oil, CBD oil, minced garlic, cumin, and sea salt. Once again, pulse the food processor for a minute, scraping down the sides halfway through.
3. Open the can of chickpeas and drain the liquid off. Add half of the can to the food processor and pulse it for 1 minute. Scrape down the sides of the bowl, then add the remaining chickpeas, and pulse for another 1 to 2 minutes.
4. Scrape down the sides, add the roasted peppers, and pulse for another 1 to 2 minutes. If the consistency of the hummus is too thick, you can always add 1 or 2 tablespoons of water.
5. Taste the hummus for salt, and then store in the refrigerator for up to one week. Enjoy!

Spicy Lime Guacamole

Whether you are looking for a snack, topping for your favorite tacos, or an appetizer, this guacamole will please a crowd! This guacamole isn't overly spicy, as the seeds of the jalapeno are removed. However, if you want to kick it up a notch, leave in the seeds and it will be even better for all you spicy food lovers.

Servings: 4
Prep time: 5 minutes
Cooking time: 0 minutes

Calories: 201 kcal
Fat: 14.8g
Protein: 2.4g
Carbs: 11g
Net Carbs: 4.7g

Ingredients:

- Avocados – 2

- CBD oil – 1 tablespoon

- Jalapeno, seeds removed and minced – 1

- Roma tomato, diced – 1

- Lime juice – 1 tablespoon

- Onion, diced – .25 cup

- Cilantro, chopped – .25 cup

- Sea salt – .5 teaspoon

Instructions:

1. In a small mixing bowl, mash the avocado using a fork and mix in the CBD oil.
2. Add in the minced jalapeno, diced Roma tomato, diced onion, chopped cilantro, lime juice, and sea salt. Enjoy with your favorite chips!

Home-Style Ranch Dressing

Whether you are looking to enjoy a hearty salad or are simply looking to enjoy a side of veggies, this home-style ranch dressing will be more flavorful than anything out of a bottle.

Servings: 6
Prep time: 3 minutes
Cooking time: 0 minutes

Calories: 72 kcal
Fat: 7g
Protein: 0.3g
Carbs: 1g
Net Carbs: 1g

Ingredients:

- Mayonnaise – .25 cup

- Buttermilk – .25 cup

- Sour cream – .25 cup

- CBD oil – 1 tablespoon

- Lemon juice – 1.5 teaspoons

- Dill, dried – .5 teaspoon

- Onion powder – .12 teaspoon

- Sea salt – .25 teaspoon

- Parsley, dried – .25 teaspoon

- Chives, dried – .25 teaspoon

- Garlic powder – .25 teaspoon
- Black pepper, ground – to taste

Instructions:

1. Whisk together the sour cream and CBD oil. Add in the mayonnaise and the buttermilk and continue to whisk until smooth.
2. Add in the herbs, lemon juice, onion powder, garlic powder, and the black pepper.
3. Taste and adjust the seasonings to your taste or preference. Enjoy!

Refreshing Italian Pasta Salad

This Italian pasta salad is styled after a traditional antipasto salad, complete with fresh mozzarella, roasted peppers, olives, salami, and more. Whether you are serving this as a side or a complete meal, it is sure to please a crowd.

Servings: 8
Prep time: 10 minutes
Cooking time: 17 minutes

Calories: 585 kcal
Fat: 35g
Protein: 17g
Carbs: 21.3g
Net Carbs: 19.7g

Ingredients:

- Pasta of choice – 1 pound

- Hard salami, chopped – 1 cup

- Mozzarella balls – 12 ounces

- Black olives, sliced – 3.8 ounces

- Red onion, diced - .5 cup

- Roasted red peppers, from a jar, chopped - .75 cup

- Cherry tomatoes, sliced in half – 2 cups

- Parsley, chopped - .25 cup

- Extra virgin olive oil - .5 cup

- CBD oil – 2 tablespoons

- Red wine vinegar - .5 cup

- Sea salt - .5 teaspoon (plus extra)

- Honey – 1 tablespoon

- Garlic, minced – 3 cloves

- Italian seasoning, dried – 1 tablespoon

Instructions:

1. Boil a large pot of water over medium heat, salt it, and then add in the pasta. Cook it until the pasta is softened but still has a bit of bite (*al dente*). This usually takes an average of 6 to 8 minutes. Drain the pasta using a colander, and then rinse it with cold water. Shake off the excess water from the pasta. Place the cooked pasta in a large bowl.

2. While the pasta boils, prepare the vinaigrette by whisking together the CBD oil and the extra virgin olive oil. Add in

the red wine vinegar, sea salt, honey, minced garlic, and Italian seasoning. Whisk the ingredients together until fully combined.

3. Add the sliced cherry tomatoes, chopped hard salami, chopped roasted red peppers, diced red onion, chopped parsley, sliced olives, and the mozzarella balls into the pasta bowl. Toss all of the ingredients with the vinaigrette.

4. Taste the Italian pasta salad and add any extra salt, if needed. Enjoy!

Black Bean Quinoa Bowls

These black bean quinoa bowls are perfect for Meatless Monday. Plus, they are full of plenty of healthy nutrients, vegetables, and whole-grains. Better yet, the quinoa and vegetable mixtures can be made ahead of time. This will give you a healthy and filling dinner to eat complete with CBD any day of the week.

Servings: 4
Prep time: 15 minutes
Cooking time: 30 minutes

Calories: 834 kcal
Fat: 31.5g
Protein: 15.7g
Carbs: 36g
Net Carbs: 28.7g

Ingredients:

- Quinoa – 1 cup

- Extra virgin olive oil – .25 cup, plus 1 tablespoon

- CBD oil – 4 teaspoons

- Red onion, diced – .5 cup

- Black beans, cooked – 30 ounces

- Garlic, minced – 2 cloves

- Cilantro, chopped – .25 cup

- Lettuce, shredded – 1 cup

- Lime juice – .25 cup

- Lime zest – 1 teaspoon

- Chili powder – .25 teaspoon

- Cayenne pepper – to taste

- Sea salt – 1.5 teaspoon

- Sharp cheddar cheese, grated – 1 cup

- Tomato, diced – 1 cup

- Avocado, sliced – 1

Instructions:

1. Place the uncooked quinoa in a metal sieve and thoroughly rinse and drain.
2. Place the quinoa, along with 2 cups of water, in a pot and bring to a boil. Reduce the heat to a simmer and cover the pot. Allow it to cook until it becomes tender and all of the liquid has been absorbed. This should take about 20 minutes.
3. Over medium heat, sauté the diced red onion in 1 tablespoon of oil until it softens, about 5 minutes. Add in the minced garlic and allow it to become fragrant but

watch it carefully so that it doesn't burn. This should take an additional minute.

4. Add the cooked black beans to the pan of onions, along with the half cup of water, chopped cilantro, cayenne pepper, and chili powder. Allow the pan to simmer until most of the liquid has cooked off, about 15 minutes. Add lime juice and season with sea salt.

5. Once the quinoa is cooked, remove it from the heat and fluff it with a fork.

6. In a small bowl, combine the remaining olive oil with the CBD oil, and stir it into the quinoa along with the lime zest.

7. Divide the quinoa between four bowls, top them with lettuce, the bean-onion mixture, diced tomato, sliced avocado, and shredded cheddar cheese. Enjoy!

Tarragon Chicken Salad

This delicious tarragon chicken is perfect for a healthy high-protein meal. The grapes add a sweet touch to the earthy tarragon and CBD, with just a hint of lemon to freshen it up. Whether you choose to serve it on crackers or bread, this tarragon chicken salad is a hit.

Servings: 4
Prep time: 5 minutes
Cooking time: 0 minutes

Calories: 208 kcal
Fat: 4g
Protein: 21.7g
Carbs: 7.3g
Net Carbs: 6.9g

Ingredients:

- Cooked chicken, chopped – 2 cups

- Grapes, chopped – 1 cup

- Celery, chopped – .25 cup

- Mayonnaise – 3 tablespoons

- Sour cream – 2 tablespoons

- lemon juice – 1 teaspoon

- CBD oil – 1 tablespoon

- Tarragon, fresh – 2 tablespoons

- Sea salt – to taste

Instructions:

1. In a medium bowl, combine the CBD oil into the sour cream. Add the mayonnaise, lemon juice, tarragon, and sea salt.
2. Then, add the chopped chicken, grapes, and celery. Enjoy on crackers or your favorite bread!

Banana Cream Chia Pudding

Whether you desire a healthy breakfast, snack, or dessert, this pudding will give you a sweet treat that will please even the picky eaters! To make it even more special, try adding some mini chocolate chips or coconut to the top.

Servings: 2
Prep time: 10 minutes
Cooking time: 0 minutes

Calories: 418 kcal
Fat: 23.7g
Protein: 6.5g
Carbs: 48g
Net Carbs: 36g

Ingredients:

- Chia seeds – .25 cup

- Coconut milk, full fat – .5 cup

- Honey – 1 tablespoon

- Almond milk – .5 cup

- Bananas – 2

- Cinnamon – 1 teaspoon

- CBD oil – .5 teaspoon

- Coconut oil, melted – 1 teaspoon

Instructions:

1. Mash one of the bananas and combine it with the melted coconut oil and the CBD oil. Add the coconut milk, honey, almond milk, and cinnamon in a bowl.
2. Cover the bowl and allow it to set in the fridge for an hour.
3. Dice the remaining banana and serve it on top of the chia pudding. Enjoy!

Chewy Nutty Brownies

No recipe section for edibles would be complete without a brownie recipe. After all, who doesn't love a good chewy brownie?

Servings: 6
Prep time: 7 minutes
Cooking time: 20 minutes

Calories: 317 kcal
Fat: 15g
Protein: 4g
Carbs: 45g
Net Carbs: 43g

Ingredients:

- Cocoa powder – .33 cup

- CBD – 1 tablespoon

- Sea salt – .5 teaspoon

- White sugar – 1 cup

- Light olive oil – .5 cup

- All-purpose flour – .5 cup

- Eggs – 2

- Vanilla extract – 1 teaspoon

- Walnuts, chopped – .33 cup (optional)

- Baking powder – .25 teaspoon

Instructions:

1. In a medium-sized metal mixing bowl, combine the light olive oil and the CBD oil. Add in the white sugar, eggs, and vanilla extract.
2. In the same bowl, add in the cocoa powder, sea salt, all-purpose flour, chopped walnuts, and baking powder. Mix just until fully combined.
3. Pour the chewy nutty brownie batter into an oil-greased 9" x 9" baking pan and bake them in a preheated oven. Bake them until a toothpick inserted in the middle of the pan comes out clean, about 20 minutes at 350° F.

Chewy Molasses Ginger Cookies

These chewy molasses ginger cookies are perfect for a cold evening by the fire, the holidays, or when you are ill and need something to settle an upset stomach. No matter what the reason or season is, these chewy molasses ginger cookies are a delicious treat.

Servings: 20
Prep time: 7 minutes
Cooking time: 20 minutes

Calories: 148 kcal
Fat: 10g
Protein: 2g
Carbs: 14g
Net Carbs: 13.4g

Ingredients:

- Butter, softened – .75 cup

- CBD oil – 1 tablespoon

- All-purpose flour – 2 cups

- Molasses – .25 cup

- Black pepper, ground – .25 teaspoon

- Eggs – 1

- White sugar – 1 cup

- Ginger, ground – 1 teaspoon

- Baking soda – 2 teaspoons

- Sea salt – .5 teaspoon

- Cloves, ground – .5 cup

- Cinnamon, ground – 1 teaspoon

Instructions:

1. Using a hand mixer, beat together the softened butter and the CBD oil. Add in the molasses, sugar, and egg.
2. In another bowl, combine the all-purpose flour, ground black pepper, ginger, cloves, cinnamon, baking soda, and sea salt.
3. Fold the dry ingredients into the butter mixture. Chill in the fridge for an hour.
4. Remove the cookies from the fridge, roll them evenly into 20 balls of dough, and bake them on a pan lined with parchment until the edges begin to set. This should take 8 to 10 minutes in an oven at 350° F.
5. Remove the cookies from the oven and allow them to cool on a wire rack. Enjoy!

Old-Fashioned Oat Cookies

These old-fashioned style oatmeal cookies are perfect for everyone. Whether or not you like chocolate, there are plenty of dessert CBD options! While these cookies are delicious on their own, you can always add raisins or chocolate chips, if you like.

Servings: 12
Prep time: 10 minutes
Cooking time: 10 minutes

Calories: 169 kcal
Fat: 5g
Protein: 4g
Carbs: 31g
Net Carbs: 29g

Ingredients:

- Butter, softened – .5 cup

- Brown sugar, packed – .33 cups

- Rolled oats – 1 cup

- Baking powder – .12 teaspoon

- White sugar – .5 cup

- All-purpose flour – 1 cup

- Egg, large – 1

- Cinnamon, ground – 1 teaspoon

- CBD oil – 1 tablespoon

- Vanilla extract – 2 teaspoons

- Baking soda – .75 teaspoon

- Nutmeg, ground – .12 teaspoon

- Sea salt – .25 teaspoon

Instructions:

1. In a medium-sized metal mixing bowl, combine the butter and CBD oil with a hand beater. Add in the brown sugar, white sugar, egg, and vanilla. Mix completely.
2. In a separate medium bowl, combine the rolled oats, baking powder, all-purpose flour, cinnamon, baking soda, nutmeg, and sea salt.
3. Add the dry ingredients to the wet ingredients and fold all of them together until combined.
4. Scoop the oat cookie dough into 12 portions onto a baking sheet lined with parchment paper and bake until the edges begin to set. About 8 to 10 minutes in a preheated oven at 350° F.
5. Remove the old-fashioned oat cookies from the pan and gently place them on a cooling rack. Enjoy!

Chocolate Chunk Macadamia Cookies

Who doesn't love chocolate chip cookies? These are taken to the next level with chunks rather than chips, macadamia nuts, and of course, CBD oil. Whether you are enjoying your cookies at home while watching a movie, on the road, or—let's admit it—the dough straight out of a bowl, you will love these!

Servings: 12
Prep time: 10 minutes
Cooking time: 10 minutes

Calories: 287 kcal
Fat: 15g
Protein: 3.5g
Carbs: 35g
Net Carbs: 33g

Ingredients:

- Brown sugar – .5 cup

- Baking soda – .5 teaspoon

- White sugar – .5 cup

- All-purpose flour – 1.5 cups

- CBD oil – 1 tablespoon

- Water, hot – 1 teaspoon

- Butter – .5 cup

- Eggs – 1 egg

- Vanilla extract – 1 teaspoon

- Salt – .25 teaspoon

- Chocolate chunks – .75 cup

- Macadamia nuts, chopped – .5 cup (optional)

Instructions:

1. In a medium-sized metal bowl, whip together the butter and CBD oil. Add in the egg, white sugar, and brown sugar. Then, add in the vanilla.
2. Combine the hot water and baking soda, and then add it to the wet ingredients.

3. In a separate medium bowl, combine the all-purpose flour, sea salt, chocolate chunks, and chopped macadamia nuts. Fold the dry ingredients into the wet ingredients.

4. Scoop the cookies into 12 even portions onto a baking sheet lined with parchment paper, leaving at least 2 inches between each cookie.

5. Bake the chocolate chunk macadamia cookies until the edges begin to golden, about 10 minutes at 350° F.

6. Remove the cookies from the oven and place on a cooling rack. Enjoy!

Peanut Butter Chocolate Cups

We all have times that we are craving a bit of chocolate, and these chocolate peanut butter cups perfectly pair with the CBD oil. Nearly everyone's' favorite pairing is chocolate and peanut butter, so why not enjoy that while getting your daily dose of CBD? Whether you are new to CBD edibles or already well-acquainted, you will love these sweet cups.

Servings: 6
Prep time: 10 minutes
Cooking time: 0 minutes

Calories: 297 kcal
Fat: 16g
Protein: 3.6g
Carbs: 23g
Net Carbs: 21g

Ingredients:

- Creamy natural peanut butter – .5 cup

- Semisweet chocolate chips – 6 ounces

- Powdered sugar – 2 tablespoons

- Sea salt – .25 teaspoon

- Vanilla extract – .25 teaspoon

- CBD oil – 1 tablespoon

Instructions:

1. In the microwave, melt the chocolate chips in the increment 30 to 45 seconds. Stir in half of the CBD oil.
2. In a small bowl, stir together the creamy peanut butter, powdered sugar, sea salt, vanilla extract, and the remaining half of the CBD oil.
3. Line 6 silicone baking cups with half of the chocolate. Set it in the freezer for a couple of minutes and allow it to set.
4. Divide the peanut butter mixture between the 6 cups, and then top it off with the remainder of the chocolate. Allow the chocolate to set in the freezer for a couple more minutes before serving. Enjoy!

Lemon Cheesecake Fat Bombs

These lemon cheesecake fat bombs are perfect for an energy boost or when you need a little snack. They offer all the flavor of lemon cheesecake, but without all the time and hassle required. Easily keep them stored in the fridge, and you can enjoy one whenever you have a craving.

Servings: 15
Prep time: 7 minutes

Cooking time: 0 minutes

Calories: 73 kcal
Fat: 7.8g
Protein: 0.7g
Carbs: 4g
Net Carbs: 4g

Ingredients:

- Cream cheese, room temperature – 6 ounces

- CBD oil – 1 tablespoon

- Lemon juice – 2 tablespoons

- Butter, softened – 4 tablespoons

- Lemon zest – 1 tablespoon

- White sugar – .25 cup

Instructions:

1. Whip together the butter and the CBD oil. Add in the cream cheese and continue to whip until light and fluffy.
2. Add in the white sugar, lemon juice, and lemon zest until fully combined.
3. Divide the lemon cream cheese mixture between 15 small silicone molds. Allow them to sit in the freezer for 10 minutes or until set.
4. Remove the lemon cheesecake fat bombs from the molds and place them in a container, which you need to store in the fridge. Enjoy!

Conclusion

Whether you are one of the many people seeking healing, pain relief, or management of a chronic illness, or you simply wish to increase your quality of life and reduce the risk of developing diseases later on, CBD can help. This powerful plant has been used medicinally for over 4,000 years. Not only has there been many amazing testimonies of management and healing of disease during this time, but clinical studies have even proven many of these benefits.

Starting out a new treatment may be scary; after all, we all know when starting a new prescription drug that it comes with a list of side effects a mile long. Even, non-prescription drugs such as aspirin have their own fair share of negatives! But, study after study has been conducted on the safety of CBD, both that derived from hemp and derived from cannabis. These studies have all concluded that it is generally safe and well-tolerated. In the case of side effects, they are generally mild. There is nothing to be afraid of when beginning CBD, especially if you first discuss it with your doctor.

No matter the method you choose to administer your CBD, whether sublingually, vaping, consuming through edibles, topically, or even capsules, you can easily and safely experience the benefits that CBD has to offer. Now that you know the tricks and tips in picking out the perfect brand and finding your dosage, there is nothing that holds you back.

Why wait any longer? You have all the knowledge you need to greatly improve your health and increase your quality of life. You won't just experience these benefits now, but well into your future as well. Find the brand and product that works for you and enjoy the gift of better health.

Made in the USA
Middletown, DE
02 November 2023

41815015R00060